D1528111

PROTECTING YOUR HEALTH WITH PROBIOTICS

The "friendly" bacteria

by George Weber, Ph.D.

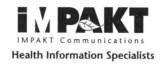

IMPAKT Communications
Health Information Specialists

www.impakt.com

Published by:
IMPAKT Communications, Inc.
P.O. Box 12496
Green Bay, WI 54307-2496
Phone: (920) 434-3838
Fax: (920) 434-8884
E-mail: info@impakt.com
www.impakt.com

Dedication

This book is dedicated to Dr. Richard Parker, the true father of the probiotics concept and my mentor in this area. He taught me the philosophy of science. He and I had years together to work and talk about the "whys and hows" of cultures. He was an exceptionally practical scientist, not swayed by either his scientific peers or his business associates. We lost him to prostate cancer in 1999, and I miss him.

—Dr. George Weber

Acknowledgements

Explaining the concept of probiotics can be challenging. It has been my goal to provide readers with scientific information in an understandable format. To do this, I relied on a team of talented individuals whom I would like to thank:

- The publisher, Karolyn A. Gazella, the editor, Frances E. FitzGerald, and the entire staff of IMPAKT Communications, Inc.
- The staff of Wakunaga of America, especially Dr. Haru Amagase, Mitsuru Takiura, Charlie Fox, Bill Stirling, and Brenda Petesch, manufacturers of Kyo-Dophilus and Probiata.
- The many scientists who helped us understand the concept of probiotics, especially Dr. Tomotari Mitsuoka, who wrote the foreword for this book.
- To my family who has supported me throughout this process.

I are grateful for this opportunity and hope you find this book a valuable addition to your natural health library.

Foreword
by Tomotari Mitsuoka, Ph.D.
Professor Emeritus
The University of Tokyo
world leader in probiotics research

The longevity of Bulgarians was, in part, due to ingesting large quantities of fermented milk that contained lactobacilli, according to Russian Nobel-prized biologist Metchnikoff. Since that time, the benefits of cultured milk products on human health have been demonstrated repeatedly. These effects include protection against constipation, diarrhea, colitis, high cholesterol levels, tumors, and harmful microbes.

Over the last four decades, significant advances have been made in the research of intestinal flora. It is becoming increasingly evident that intestinal flora plays a vital role in human health.

The so-called "friendly" bacteria include the lactic acid bacteria, such as bifidobacteria and lactobacilli. They produce lactic acid as the major end product during the fermentation of carbohydrates. However, they do not produce putrefactive or toxic chemicals. They are not pathogenic bacteria, either.

"Unfriendly" or bad bacteria may generate substances that threaten human health. Among these are certain putrefactive substances, including ammonia, hydrogen sulfide, amines, phenols, indoles, and secondary bile acids. These substances may damage the intestines directly, and the rest of the body indirectly. Because the substances are distributed and absorbed, they can potentially contribute to conditions such as cancer, arteriosclerosis, hypertension, liver disorders, autoimmune diseases, and immunosuppression.

Clearly, imbalanced intestinal flora contributes to disease. The greater the amount of harmful substances produced in the intestine, the more our health is threatened. The harmful effects are not apparent right away, but they will emerge eventually.

Fortunately, balanced intestinal flora appears to protect and promote health and longevity. Certain factors enhance this vital balance. They include a nutritionally well-balanced diet, and consumption of functional foods such as dietary fiber, oligosaccharides, and probiotics. These functional foods promote beneficial bacteria or suppress harmful bacteria.

Functional foods are thought to improve mental well-being and physical conditioning, as well as reduce the risk of disease. They may protect against hypertension, diabetes, cancer, high cholesterol levels, anemia, and platelet aggregation.

In 1989, Fuller coined the term "probiotics." It referred to a "live microbial feed supplement which beneficially affects the host animal by improving its intestinal microbial balance." The benefits of probiotics for human health soon became apparent. Researchers found that probiotics can alleviate lactose intolerance, lower serum cholesterol, relieve diarrhea, stimulate the immune system, control infections, suppress tumors, and protect against harmful bacteria, colon/bladder cancer, allergies, and other autoimmune diseases.

This book will focus on some of the benefits of probiotics. It will also help the reader choose the highest quality probiotic to nourish his or her health.

My greatest hope is that *Protecting Your Health With Probiotics: The "Friendly" Bacteria* will increase your understanding of this remarkable functional food and contribute to your health and well-being.

Contents

Introduction

Is it Us Against Them?

Most of us have probably seen on television commercials what bacteria look like. Some of them are not too far off. They come in a variety of shapes: short rods or spheres, sometimes growing in chains like beads on a string. Others grow in groups or even pairs. Like everything else in nature, bacteria consume material to grow and multiply. They also produce by-products, or waste. Some of these by-products can benefit the bacteria and their environment. Other by-products are regarded as defense mechanisms. These defense molecules try to protect the bacteria from harm—even if it means destroying their world, which in some cases is us!

Bacteria are everywhere. Consider this: No matter how hard we try to get rid of them, there are more bacteria in and on you than there are people on this earth. The intestines alone have about 100 trillion bacteria, which outnumber all the cells in the human body 10 to 1.

But don't be too worried. You've been living *with* them since before you could walk or talk. Most don't stay around that long. It has been estimated that humans excrete a couple of trillion bacteria through the feces every day. That's about one-third of our fecal matter.

There are more than 400 species of bacteria, many of which share your internal space every second of every day. It is quite obvious that the sheer number of bacteria can affect us profoundly. They metabolize, reproduce, and colonize just like the cells that make up our bodies. Many produce by-products and substances that can benefit us. They can mutate or change in response to their environment (our bodies) and, unfortunately, some can produce substances that are not good for us. However, you will discover that it goes both ways—not only do the bacteria influence us, but we also influence our internal bacterial population. It's only when we ignore them—or ignore that they even exist—that we can get into serious trouble. Hopefully, this book will help prevent that.

In our fight for optimum health, we need to recognize that some strains of bacteria are serious adversaries. In fact, Joshua Lederberg, who won the 1958 Nobel Prize for his work in bacterial genetics, stated: "...people are the underdogs in any battle with microbes. Their sheer number and speed of replication give them a decided edge against human beings."

We may be the underdogs, but we can still conquer the bad bacteria, and keep and enhance the good bacteria.

No need to panic

Yes, the numbers are overwhelming. And yes, the magnitude of bacteria is unfathomable. However, there is no need to throw in the towel.

As with most compelling battles, there are good guys and bad guys. The bad bacteria can lead to a variety of illnesses. Some are merely irritating, such as temporary gas or bloating, and others more life-threatening. Depending on where they eventually reside, these harmful bacteria can lead to a variety of maladies, including:
- Diarrhea and constipation
- Infections
- Ulcers
- Food poisoning
- Irritable bowel syndrome
- Colitis
- Vaginitis and candidiasis
- The typical "sore throat"
- A weakened immune system
- Serious bacterial/toxin infections that can even result in death.

An estimated 20 million people in the United States are afflicted with ailments of the gastrointestinal tract. These include ulcers, hepatitis, hernias, and cancer of the esophagus. Gastrointestinal diseases are also responsible for 30 percent of cancer deaths; 25 percent of operations, excluding tonsillectomies; 10 percent of the total days that adults are ill; and $17 billion in direct healthcare costs.

Most of us have heard the terms "salmonella" or "*E. coli.*" These are names of bacteria that are commonly associated with contaminated food and water, which can lead to a variety of mysterious symptoms and hard-to-diagnose conditions. The Center for Disease Control and Prevention (CDC) has estimated that approximately 76 million cases of food-borne illnesses occur each year, leading to 325,000 hospitalizations and over 5,000 deaths. The estimated cost is over 30 billion dollars. But most of us, when we're afflicted, don't think that our discomfort is worth a call to the CDC. So, the figures are actually underestimated.

Truly, we "are what we eat." When we inadvertently eat the wrong things, we can be subjected to a wide variety of gastrointestinal discomforts. In addition, people don't just have "an upset stomach" without other associated symptoms such as a headache, anxiety, and loss of appetite. However, there is hope.

The realization that both good and bad bacteria have always been around us has intrigued scientists for years. However, differentiating between the two can be difficult. There is a simple microbiology maxim that states: Any microorganism outside of its natural environment should be considered a pathogen. What does this mean? Simple. The bacteria that normally reside on your skin, for example, are just fine residing there. But if they happen to get into your bloodstream by way of a cut or scrape, they could be the beginning of a serious infection. Likewise, if we inhale or breathe in air that contains a large number of flu viruses, depending on our immune system at the time, we could get the flu. The same applies to eating and drinking. Ingesting food or drink that is "contaminated" with bacteria could result in some of the things previously mentioned.

We can't become paranoid about it, however. After all, how can people fight things they can't see? Walk around in a sterile environment? Eat sterile food? Breathe sterile air? Hardly. We weren't built to be that way. In actuality, we were designed to coexist with all these microorganisms. They were here long before we even knew they existed and they'll be here long after we're gone.

Joshua Lederberg says we're the underdogs when we fight them. But let's face it, they don't have brains and we're a lot bigger! We can't live life wondering whether everything we touch, eat, drink, or breathe will make us sick. There are ways you can stack the cards in your favor.

In my discussions of a balance of good and bad bacteria, I'm not talking about a 50-50 split. It's not that we're normally walking around with half "good" bacteria and half "bad" bacteria. It's normally heavily weighted to the "good" side. By how much? We honestly don't know. What we do know is that in the midst of the billions and billions of bacteria that are typically in our gastrointestinal tract, as little as a few hundred of the really nasty ones can cause life-threatening illness. Protecting ourselves from these and the other minor players can be enhanced by supplementing with the ones we know are good for us—the probiotics.

To help alleviate the symptoms and conditions that bad bacteria can cause, we need enough good bacteria. Also known as the "friendly" bacteria, probiotics are the good bacteria. They help replenish the good bacteria in our systems so we stay healthy. Probiotics produce a variety of compounds, including natural lactic acids, that help inhibit the growth of the "bad" bacteria, thereby blocking them from gaining a foothold and causing illness.

The complex balance of bacteria in your body, in conjunction with your immune system and other important body functions, determines, in many cases, whether you are to be healthy or unhealthy. There must always be enough of the good bacteria to offset the potential negative effects of the bad. This book will discuss, in detail, how to achieve and maintain a healthy balance.

I will begin by explaining how the gastrointestinal system works and its importance to overall health. From there, you will learn what probiotics are and how human strain probiotics can help prevent and even treat illness; specific conditions that can benefit from probiotic use; and how to safely and effectively use probiotics.

Probiotics can have a far-reaching impact on your health. They provide protection in a toxic world. They help restore internal balance that not only protects against illness but promotes optimal health and vitality. Best of all, probiotic supplements are effective, safe, and easy to incorporate into your daily health regimen.

The probiotics plan

Henry David Thoreau wrote: "Nature is doing her best to keep us healthy."

The good bacteria inside you are critical for your good health. The probiotics plan ensures that you always have an ample supply of the good bacteria.

The most effective health-promoting program includes:
• Maintaining good sanitary surroundings;
• A healthful diet;
• Regular exercise; and
• Attention to the mind/body connection.

When you incorporate probiotics into this comprehensive health plan, you will be doing your best to carry out what nature intended...keeping yourself healthy.

The process begins with proper digestion. Unfortunately, poor digestion has become a major problem in North America. It has been estimated that about 70 million Americans suffer from some type of digestion problem. Gas, bloating, diarrhea, constipation, and even skin conditions can all be signs of digestive disturbances.

However, digestive problems have gone beyond the irritating and moved into the danger zone. As long ago as 1987, the problem was evident, with 13 percent of all hospitalizations due to digestive issues. In 1992, the United States population spent $107 billion fighting digestive diseases. According to the CDC, nearly 35 million visits to the emergency room in 1997 were due to diseases of the digestive system.

The prescription and over-the-counter drug industry has jumped into action to take advantage of this growing problem. They continue to introduce dozens of new digestive remedies—most of which simply alleviate symptoms without addressing the underlying cause.

Yes, digestive problems have reached near epidemic proportions. It's not surprising that scientific, as well as consumer interest in probiotics is booming. Probiotic supplements have been shown, in both laboratory and clinical studies, to help alleviate many of the problems associated with digestive disorders. They can help restore harmony to the internal environment, which is often in disarray.

But before we explore the power of probiotics, it is important to understand the workings of the digestive system.

Chapter One

Understanding Digestion

An ecosystem is "an ecological community together with its environment, functioning as a unit." Scientists have called the digestive system, "…the most complex ecosystem known."

How can that be, you ask? It's just a stomach and some intestines, right? From a simplistic perspective, that may be true. However, a sophisticated community of microflora (i.e., bacteria) inhabit the human digestive system, which is 400 square meters. How big is 400 square meters? Imagine placing your digestive system on the ground in front of you. It would cover the size of a tennis court! And remember, it is populated with more bacteria than there are people on the earth.

To better understand bacteria and their implications on health, you need to understand the important functions of the digestive system. However, before I begin my discussion of the digestive system, let's define some terminology:

- The digestive system represents the tract from the mouth to the anus, and everything in between.
- The gastrointestinal tract (GI), on the other hand, refers to just the stomach and intestines.
- The intestines are also referred to as the "gut."
- The first part of the small intestine from the stomach is known as the duodenum.
- The large intestine is also known as the colon.

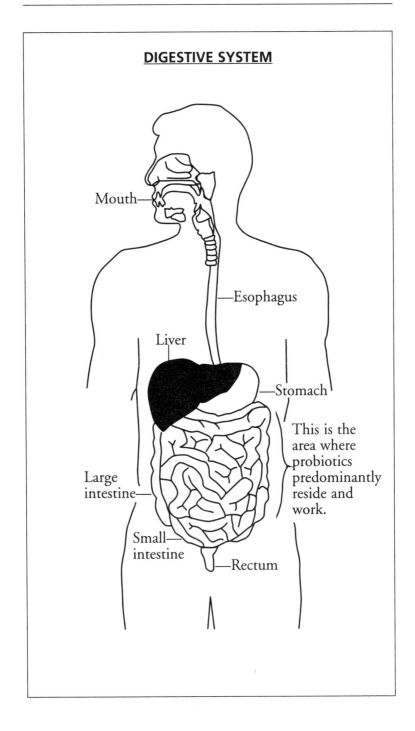

DIGESTIVE SYSTEM

Mouth

Esophagus

Liver

Stomach

This is the area where probiotics predominantly reside and work.

Large intestine

Small intestine

Rectum

The digestive system is a very active, ever-changing environment. Even as you read this sentence, bacteria are moving and morphing inside of you at an unbelievable pace.

Among the hundreds of different species of bacteria, there are many different genetic variations. Why? In order for our bodies to survive and thrive in varying environments, the digestive ecosystem needs to be diverse and adaptable.

That's an important point. Hundreds of different species of bacteria, with many variations, are constantly evolving, colonizing, and moving throughout the digestive system. It is this flurry of activity that makes the digestive system so complex. Good bacteria help our inside environment adapt to outside environmental factors, including diet, stress, climate, and toxins in our air and water. For example, your internal bacterial community will react differently whether you live in Alaska versus Hawaii, or whether you are a meat-eater or a vegetarian.

The human body is truly amazing. Consider what will happen if we are forced through necessity or climate, for example, to live on a specific kind of food that we can't easily digest. The make-up of our internal microflora will change to produce the enzymes needed to help us extract the nutrients we need from that food.

Our internal community of friendly bacteria help us survive and thrive in varying environments. However, if the unfriendly bacteria establish themselves in the digestive system and are allowed to produce toxic by-products, the internal environment may rapidly start to fail. The results can range from mild to devastating.

Under extreme conditions, bacterial toxins can be released into the bloodstream, and they can then make their way to any part of the body. That's why bacterial imbalance can have profound, far-reaching, negative effects on our health. Conversely, digestive harmony can help us maintain optimal health and avoid illness.

Digesting the facts

The purpose of the digestive system is really three-fold:

1. To pull nutrients from the foods we eat.
2. To digest these nutrients so they can be absorbed and utilized by the body.
3. To eliminate the harmful by-products, bad bacteria, and waste that are left over.

Our digestive system is the first and last contact we have with the foods we eat. This is important when you consider that without proper nourishment, we will die. And without proper digestion, we don't have proper nourishment.

From the moment the food touches your tongue, it will go through a variety of changes before it is eliminated as waste. Digestion chemically and mechanically breaks down the foods we eat into an absorbable, usable form. Salt, simple sugars, and water can be absorbed as they are; however, starches, fats, proteins, and complex sugars must be broken down to gain their nutritive value.

The mechanical process of chewing starts the digestive process by breaking down the food and mixing it with enzymes in the saliva. In our society, we tend to rush this process and not chew food thoroughly. This is unfortunate, because chewing food completely is an important first step toward optimum digestion.

The food then travels down the esophagus to the stomach. In the stomach, the digestive process continues with a chemical reaction of enzymes and hydrochloric acid. After the material is blended with gastric juices, it is further transported to the small intestines to continue the digestive process. A highly acidic stomach is preferred, as it will ensure proper breakdown of foods. Low stomach acid can lead to bloating and gas, common conditions in the United States today.

"The stomach provides the perfect surroundings in which pepsin (an enzyme that works on proteins) can do its job, and also kills off many antigens," explains Kenneth Bock, M.D., in his book *The Road to Immunity.* "Only the most durable microorganisms survive the passage through an optimally acidified stomach."

The mushy substance created in the stomach, known as chyme, is then sent to the small intestine. The pancreas secretes more enzymes and juices, including carbohydrate-digesting enzymes (amylase), protein-digesting enzymes (trypsin), and fat-digesting enzymes (lipase). The pancreas also secretes bicarbonate to achieve a less acidic environment and optimum pH level.

While the stomach needs to be more acidic to break down the food, the intestine needs to be more alkaline to start removing nutrients from the food so they can be absorbed into the bloodstream. When everything is working properly in the upper digestive tract, only nutrients are absorbed into the bloodstream, while waste and unabsorbed material are eventually eliminated from the body.

After the small intestine has pulled out all the nutrients it can, it passes the nearly liquid substance to the large intestine. By this time, most of the nutrients have been taken and transported to other areas of the body. The remaining substance becomes firmer in the large intestine because the water is reabsorbed. Food will spend most of its time in the large intestine. It takes about 10 hours for the food to wind its way through the colon.

Of course, the final step of the digestive process is defecation, or release of the material from your body with a bowel movement.

There's plenty of truth to the adage, "Death begins in the colon." Supporting colon health helps safeguard overall health. Many experts agree that optimal health depends on at least one effortless bowel movement each day. Adequate amounts of fiber in the diet can help ensure this.

Necessity of dietary fiber

After carbohydrates, protein, fat, vitamins, and minerals, fiber is considered the sixth nutrient. The most critical function of dietary fiber is to push out the waste in the intestine smoothly and efficiently. Fiber is the cleaning substance of the intestine. This nutrient is unique in that it can help with both constipation and diarrhea by contributing to proper stool weight and faster transit time through our digestive system.

FIBER SOURCES

- **BAKED BEANS ($^1/_2$ CUP)**   =   **8.8 GRAMS**

- **CARROTS (1 CUP)**   =   **4.6 GRAMS**

- **BROCCOLI (1 CUP)**   =   **4.4 GRAMS**

- **LENTILS ($^1/_2$ CUP)**   =   **3.7 GRAMS**

- **APPLE (W/SKIN)**   =   **3.5 GRAMS**

- **RAISINS ($^1/_4$ CUP)**   =   **3.1 GRAMS**

- **WHEAT BREAD (2 SLICES)**   =   **2.8 GRAMS**

In addition to promoting bowel regularity, fiber slows gastric emptying. This means that food is released into the small intestine more gradually, which means blood glucose levels rise more gradually.

High fiber intake also appears to:
- Protect against cancer;
- Lower blood cholesterol and blood pressure;
- Reduce the absorption of excessive fat; and
- Protect against colon cancer.

Moreover, fiber plays a key role in intestinal bacterial balance. In order to maintain an optimal balance, it is important to eliminate the waste before bad bacteria can take over. Fiber helps reduce the population of bad bacteria, which create toxic chemicals. By regulating the balance of intestinal bacteria, fiber enhances healthy body functions.

When you combine fiber with probiotics, such as *L. acidophilus* and *Bifidobacterium*, you may greatly improve your intestinal condition, and restore a youthful intestinal bacterial balance.

Most Americans consume about 12 grams of fiber per day. According to the American Dietetic Association, we should consume from 20 to 30 grams of fiber per day. Greater than 30 grams of fiber can interfere with absorption of nutrients, interfere with medications, and potentially bind to minerals.

Bacterial colonization

The process of peristalsis is what keeps the food moving. Muscle contractions within the digestive tract squeeze the undigested food along to the next step. Throughout the process, microorganisms, including good and bad bacteria, can cling to the lining of the intestines. The ability to stick to the wall of the intestines determines whether a particular bacteria will colonize, multiply, and become a resident of the GI tract.

"Different strains compete for space and, just to make things more interesting, various types of epithelial cells at different sites have striking differences in how suitable they are for the adherence of individual kinds of bacteria," writes Dr. Bock. "This helps explain why different bacteria colonize different parts of the GI tract." Yeast, for example, has a greater chance of "sticking" to the lining of the colon and vagina versus other parts of the body.

Interestingly, at birth, the intestinal tract is sterile and free of bacteria and fungi. Within a month or so, bacteria similar to adults have formed in the infant's evolving digestive system, starting with those first introduced if the child is nursing. From there, the complex digestive ecosystem develops, based on both outside and inside influences. It is during this early developmental stage that attention should be paid to maintaining optimum bacterial balance.

What happens when the microbial population of the normal GI tract is under attack? The body suffers through a rebuilding phase as the good bacteria try to rebound. This occurs naturally but can be a slow process. You can struggle with bacterial imbalance symptoms, such as fatigue, for weeks or even months before an ideal balance has been re-established.

Importance of enzymes

The entire process of digestion would come to a screeching halt if it weren't for enzymes. Presently, more than 3,000 different types of enzymes have been identified, with millions of them circulating throughout the body. Their effects on human health are profound. No plant, animal, or human could exist without enzymes. All of our body functions are based upon enzyme reactions in our body/cells. Specific enzymes also come into play throughout the process of digestion. As soon as food enters your mouth, it is greeted by enzymes in the saliva. Enzymes are the front-line laborers of the digestive construction crew. Like jackhammers, they bust apart food into smaller pieces so it can then be absorbed and used by the body. As mentioned previously, there are three main types of enzymes on this crew:

1. Amylases, which break down carbohydrates.
2. Lipases, which break down fats.
3. Proteases, which break down proteins.

Without these and other enzymes, the body would not be able to digest, and most importantly utilize, fats, proteins, carbohydrates, vitamins, minerals, and other important nutrients from our foods. Without the ability to utilize these food substances, our food is not really "feeding" us at all—it is literally just going in one end and out the other.

A deficiency or absence of a certain enzyme could lead to improper digestion. The result may be a wide range of symptoms.

Enzymes are critical workers within the complex digestive system. Not only should you take steps to ensure you have the right balance of enzymes in your body, you should also take steps to enhance their effectiveness.

Enzyme supplements are available over-the-counter at health food stores and pharmacies. Some supplements contain key enzymes, including protease, lipase, and amylase, along with probiotics such as *Lactobacillus acidophilus*.

One of the more common enzymes that many of us have difficulty with is the one responsible for the digestion of lactose, the sugar found in milk. Probiotics can help surmount this difficulty. This will be discussed in greater detail in a later chapter.

Digestive disturbances

Now that you know how the digestive system works, you can see why it is so important to promote digestive harmony. It is nearly impossible for the vast number of intestinal bacteria and their extremely rapid rate of growth not to have a significant impact on our health—either contributing to that harmony or causing chaos.

Clearly, one of the most influential aspects of the digestive ecosystem is the battle between good and bad bacteria. Controlling the bad by outnumbering them with the good is a strategy proven to be successful.

Hundreds of bacteria compete for the same positions within your digestive system. Both good and bad bacteria have the same objective, which is to survive by any means possible and secure a prime location(s) in your intestines.

Quality probiotic supplements can supply you with friendly bacteria to reduce the space left to which the bad bacteria can adhere. The more friendly inhabitants you have, the better off you are.

What happens when the bad make their presence known? Illness sets in. It can be subtle at first—possibly a slight case of diarrhea or constipation with a dull headache. Then it may escalate.

Yet your body is sophisticated enough to provide you with the information you need to make decisions about your health. It does this in the form of symptoms. Most of these symptoms are subtle at first. On those days when you just "don't feel like yourself" or you think you are "fighting something," it may be that the bad bacteria are taking over. That's when you need to pay attention. Don't wait for something more serious to develop. Probiotic supplements can help you prevent those sick days, or help reduce their frequency.

Chapter Two

Powerful Probiotics

Probiotics are friendly bacteria that can become powerful allies in our fight for vitality and good health. Probiotics are those special bacteria that scientists have studied for decades. The definition of probiotics is: beneficial organisms that help improve the environment of the intestinal tract. That makes perfect sense. After all, the Greek term "pro" means "for," and "bio" means "life."

Probiotics work like recycling plants that transform waste products from the environment into useful items. These small probiotic factories are designed to produce good bacteria molecules. High-quality probiotic supplements deliver billions of living human strain organisms that are designed to live in the digestive system (see p. 39). When they reach their targeted destination, these friendly bacteria will help fortify the body's internal environment and, therefore, contribute to our overall health and vitality.

How it all began

The concept of probiotics is not new. In fact, at the turn of the 20th century, the idea of probiotics was so important that it earned microbiologist Eli Metchnikoff a Nobel Prize. Metchnikoff believed that some bacteria produced toxins in the intestines that encouraged disease and shortened life. Conversely, he felt that probiotics were the elixir of life.

Metchnikoff believed that good bacteria such as *Lactobacillus acidophilus* could overpower bad bacteria if they became the dominant player in the intestine.

For years, the claim that friendly bacteria could actually prevent illness was discounted as unscientific folklore. Nearly a century later, however, a substantial and growing body of scientific evidence supports Metchnikoff's theory.

In the mid-1970s, studies involving continued feeding of animals with specially isolated strains of lactobacilli resulted in Dr. Richard B. Parker's Probiotics Concept. That was the first use of what has now become a common term. Today, probiotics are sold world-wide as dietary supplements to enhance and maintain the ratio of good to bad bacteria within the digestive system.

"Probiotic-containing products are common in Japan and Europe," wrote professor Mary Ellen Sanders in *Food Technology*, November 1999. "In the United States, probiotics are just now receiving attention by the food industry as healthful ingredients for an increasingly health-conscious consumer."

Subtle, yet powerful

The question is, however, do we really need to actually supplement the diet with these friendly bacteria?

It's true that probiotics may not provide you with an immediate and noticeable effect on your health, like aspirin, for example. Rather, the effect of taking probiotics will more likely be seen in the absence of illness and the way you feel overall.

The fact is, you may already be tipping the bacterial balance scales in favor of the bad bacteria without even knowing it. Even if you have enough friendly bacteria, if you don't nourish them with what they need, they will be ineffective.

Following are some of the key factors that can help the bad bacteria take the lead:

- **Antibiotic use.** It is now widely understood that antibiotics are indiscriminate in the type of bacteria they kill—both good and bad. We will go into more detail on this topic in the next chapter.
- **Estrogen use.** Birth control pills and prescription estrogen have been shown to disrupt normal intestinal floral balance.

- **Travel.** Any kind of trip, especially out of the country, can influence the condition of the digestive tract.
- **Stress.** Emotional and physical stress can have a profound impact on our health and bacterial balance. Pay close attention to how your GI tract responds to stress.
- **Lifestyle factors.** Lack of physical activity, low-fiber diet, negative attitude, smoking, and drinking too much alcohol and not enough fresh water, will most likely result in digestive disharmony.
- **Food- and water-borne contaminants.** This is dramatically illustrated in cases of *E. coli* breakouts in our food supply. Or, how many times have you heard the phrase, "Don't drink the water" when you travel? In addition, chemical preservatives and additives are part of the processed foods we eat.

It appears that the entire bacterial community is subject to your external actions and environment. Here are six general guidelines that will help tip the scales in your favor:

1. **Eat a healthful diet** of fruits and vegetables. Try to consume unprocessed foods free of chemicals, preservatives, and artificial flavors and colors. Also limit consumption of red meat and simple sugars.

BACTERIAL IMBALANCE

- **PHYSICAL AND EMOTIONAL STRESS**

- **UNHEALTHY LIFESTYLE CHOICES**

- **FOOD AND WATER CONTAMINANTS**

- **ANTIBIOTICS**

- **ESTROGEN**

- **TRAVEL**

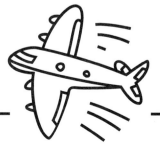

2. **Exercise consistently.**
3. **Drink at least eight, 8-ounce glasses of fresh drinking water daily.**
4. **Get adequate rest.**
5. **Try to control stress** and resolve emotional, deep-seated issues, as this has been shown to negatively affect intestinal health.
6. **Take a probiotic supplement** that contains stable, human strain bacteria.

Remember, there is a good chance that if your external body is healthy, your internal body of bacteria is also healthy and in balance.

Bacteria basics

As I have pointed out, the activities within the entire bacterial community are very complicated. Trillions of bacteria compete for space and colonizing opportunities within the complex digestive system. They all live in very close quarters and maintain a hectic pace as they complete their designated tasks. That's right, specific bacteria are more than just transient renters of GI space, they are active participants in their own working-class world. That's why it is essential to supplement the diet with human strain probiotics.

While there are hundreds of strains of bacteria, the two most common types of probiotics are *Lactobacillus acidophilus* and *Bifidobacterium*. Unfortunately, there has been much confusion over these probiotics. It is likely that the debate over the best way to use probiotics (i.e., dosage, type) will continue as the popularity and necessity of these supplements increases. The scientific community has confirmed, however, that at least 1 billion living cells is the appropriate daily dosage. Other aspects of probiotic supplementation have also been confirmed.

For instance, we know that *Lactobacillus acidophilus* is mainly found in the small intestine, while the large intestine is the primary home for *Bifidobacterium*. Both strains can make a profound contribution to our health. Maintaining high levels of both probiotics is very important; however, it's not just power in numbers. We also need to keep these friendly bacteria functioning at peak performance as consistently as possible.

Interestingly, the type of bacteria living in your system may actually be the same whether you are feeling great or lousy. How can that be? Good bacteria can work harder for you when you are healthy compared to when you are feeling tired and weak. The good bacteria may still be present, but they are just not up for the tasks at hand.

The health and magnitude of your friendly bacteria mirror your own health. What's good for you is good for them. When you eat healthful foods, get enough rest, and control stress levels, you feel great, right? The same is true for your friendly bacteria. Treat them well and they will serve you well. Deprive them of what they need and they will just take up space without making any real contribution to your health. And they certainly won't be able to compete with the bad bacteria.

"…when bifidobacteria (a probiotic) are in a good state of health, they will detoxify pollutants and carcinogens (cancer-causing substances), as well as manufacture the various B vitamins…" explains naturopathic physician Leon Chaitow of the University of Westminster, England. "When in a poor state of health, however, they just cannot do these jobs as well or at all."

Probiotics fulfill very specific tasks when they are in peak condition. These tasks are critical to your overall health. Here are just some examples of what the good bacteria can do:

- Bifidobacteria produce important B vitamins, including niacin, B6, folic acid, and biotin. Bifidobacteria are also very sensitive to their environment. Fewer bifidobacteria may dramatically affect the body's production of these B vitamins, also known as the anti-stress vitamins.
- They manufacture the enzyme lactase, which helps us digest dairy products.
- They improve digestive efficiency and encourage proper bowel function.
- They literally recycle toxins.
- They can work to reduce cholesterol levels by contributing to cholesterol metabolism and utilization.

- They stimulate a positive, powerful immune system response, not just in the GI system, but also throughout the body.
- In an effort to protect "their territory," some can even produce substances that kill or deactivate hostile disease-causing bacteria—you know, the bad guys. They can change the local levels of acidity, or deprive bad bacteria of their nutrients, or they can actually produce their own antibiotic-like substances, which can kill invading bacteria, viruses, and yeasts.

It is certainly in your best interest to keep your good bacteria in tip-top shape. In addition to keeping your friendly bacteria healthy, it is vital to keep your digestive system stocked with them. That's right, you need to keep packing them in. **The friendly, as well as the unfriendly bacteria, continuously die off and are eliminated from the body. It is vital to continually replenish your supply of good bacteria to offset the bad bacteria that make their way into your system via food, air, water, etc.**

That's why probiotic supplementation is so important. Unless you are living in a pure environment, you are being exposed to bad bacteria constantly. It is up to you to keep your friendly bacteria healthy, and help them outnumber their internal adversaries.

Probiotics can help treat a variety of illnesses. They can also be incorporated into your individual health program to help prevent these illnesses.

Remember, the most successful health program should include:
- A healthful diet.
- Consistent exercise.
- Mind/body awareness.
- Nutritional supplements, including human strain probiotics.

Chapter Three

Explore the Possibilities

While medical science has made great strides in what we call "crisis medicine" or emergency care, it seems sometimes that we lose ground in other areas. Chronic, degenerative conditions such as cancer, heart disease, arthritis, and diabetes continue to escalate, causing disability and taking millions of lives each year. Other, more "modern" illnesses, such as chronic fatigue syndrome, fibromyalgia, food allergies, and attention deficit disorder, also appear to be affecting more of our population. Emotional disorders, such as depression and anxiety, have become commonplace. Neurological diseases, such as senile dementia and Alzheimer's, previously reserved for a small group of the elderly, have now penetrated the baby-boom generation.

It is not surprising that many of us are searching for ways to prevent illness and maintain optimum health as we age. For some, the goal is simple—to achieve a high level of vitality. For others, the goal is much more serious as they battle a disease that has already taken hold.

In this chapter, we will address specific illnesses and evaluate the science supporting the use of probiotics. But before we begin with specifics, we must first evaluate the effects of probiotics on the immune system—our most powerful weapon against illness and disease.

The human immune system is an amazing blend of trillions of proactive cells. They are on duty 24 hours a day, every day, to eliminate invading organisms. When it is healthy and operating at peak capacity, the immune system can destroy many types of foreign materials, bacteria, and cancer-causing substances. However, if your immune system is not in peak condition, you may get sick. Finding ways to keep your immune system healthy, and stimulate its activity, will help you maintain or regain good health.

Probiotics and immunity

When something is systemic, it affects the entire body. When it is localized, it only affects one area. This is important because scientists have discovered that probiotics may have both a systemic and localized effect on immunity.

Within the digestive system, we have immune cells that keep that particular area of the body healthy. The digestive tract is our first line of defense in the body. And because of its size (remember the tennis court!), the gastrointestinal tract is technically the largest immune organ in the human body.

Our immune system works at our front line of defense to fight the various bacteria that enter. If this front line immune barrier is deficient, illness may occur.

The immune cells in the digestive system work hard to protect against infection and possibly even cancers of the stomach and colon. This is important, considering the impact these cancers have on our society. According to *Taber's Medical Dictionary*, 1992 estimates indicated that colon/rectal cancer was second only to breast cancer in the most frequently diagnosed cancers among women. For men, it was third, with lung and prostate number one and two, respectively.

Research has confirmed that the digestive system's immune response is related to, but still somewhat different than that of the body's overall immune system activity. While the same players (e.g., killer cells, macrophages) exist in both places, the immune cells of the digestive system work with enzymes and friendly bacteria to achieve the shared goal of getting rid of antigens (i.e., foreign substances). This localized effect has a systemic influence, meaning it helps the overall body. The immune system's team in the digestive tract helps control the antigens, thereby preventing them from becoming absorbed through the intestines to circulate throughout the body.

Enter probiotics. While we don't know exactly how probiotics help stimulate the immune system, scientific evidence has demonstrated that probiotic consumption (specifically lactobacilli) can:

- Activate immune system cells, specifically macrophages and lymphocytes;
- Increase natural killer cell activity; and
- Stimulate a systemic (i.e., general body) immune response.

While a localized immune system response is vital, it is the systemic immune response that may offer the most far-reaching benefit. For this reason, many scientists have focused their attention on this exciting field. Research in this fairly uncharted area has increased dramatically over the past decade. It is expected that the systemic immune-enhancing effects of probiotics will be scientifically confirmed.

What does this mean to you? If researchers continue to confirm that probiotics have a systemic immune effect, you can use these substances to fend off illness and keep your immune system strong.

Because of the safety of probiotics (which I will discuss in more detail in the next chapter), I believe they should be taken daily. Probiotics should be used on a consistent basis to maintain a healthy GI tract.

In cases of a weakened immune system, I also recommend that probiotics be taken with aged garlic extract to help increase T- and B-cell counts.

Antibiotics and probiotics

Undoubtedly, one of the most common ways North Americans disrupt intestinal bacterial balance is through their use of antibiotics. Antibiotics are prescription drugs principally designed and developed to kill the bacteria that cause infections and their sometimes fatal symptoms. Unfortunately, they are not as specific as we'd like to think. Although antibiotics are designed to kill specific "bad" bacteria, many of them kill specific "bad" *and* "good" kinds of bacteria. That is, most antibiotic prescriptions are specific for general classes of bacteria—not specific organisms. Consequently, to treat a bacterial infection, such as strep throat, we would take an antibiotic. It would eventually make its way to our throat via the bloodstream to attack the infection.

While the targeted bacteria is often outside of the digestive system, the antibiotic must still travel through this delicate and complex bacterial ecosystem in order to achieve its end result. Along the way, these antibiotic drugs invariably kill beneficial bacteria and disrupt our internal bacterial balance, causing numerous side effects.

Certainly, antibiotic medicines have helped millions of people and saved many lives. Individuals with strep throat, Lyme disease, and other acute bacterial infections can and do benefit greatly from antibiotics. Unfortunately, the overuse of antibiotics is causing serious problems. Often, an antibiotic is prescribed for a viral infection when, in reality, antibiotics are not effective against viruses. You know you have a virus when your doctor says, "It just needs to run its course." The common cold and influenza are two examples of common viruses.

Over-prescription of antibiotics has resulted in new bacterial strains. Simple bacteria that were easily treated decades ago with antibiotic therapy no longer respond. Because survival is of utmost importance to bacteria, these simple strains are not so simple any more. They have morphed into more complex organisms (i.e., "super germs") in order to withstand the antibiotic medicines designed to attack them. Remember, Joshua Lederberg's quote about being the underdog?

"The age of antibiotics is fast coming to a close," writes Michael Weiner, Ph.D., in his book, *Maximum Immunity*. "Because of their great numbers, viruses and bacteria have quickly evolved resistant strains for almost every major man-made pharmaceutical."

Infectious organisms, such as tuberculosis and *E. coli*, were once thought to be under control. However, they are now resurfacing and are more challenging to treat than ever before. According to Dr. Cynthia Whitney of the CDC, "It's become even more worrisome in the last two years. There are definitely some strains that are fast learners."

In an editorial in a recent issue of the *New England Journal of Medicine*, Drs. Richard P. Wenzel and Michael B. Edmond of Virginia Commonwealth University stated, "The antibiotic era is barely 60 years old, yet the inappropriate use of these drugs threatens our ability to cope with infections."

Jim Hensen, creator of the Muppets, died of a bacterial illness. There was no antibiotic treatment available because he had developed a resistance to antibiotics.

Childhood ear infections are a common example of antibiotic overuse. An estimated 90 percent of all ear infections will heal on their own without antibiotic treatment. And yet, prescription antibiotics continue to be among the most popular and widely used drugs available.

"Even if the antibiotic does not help us get well any faster, there is a tendency to want that antibiotic prescription anyway," explains children's health expert Mary Ann Block, D.O. "This attitude may have actually put our future health in jeopardy." Dr. Block explains that giving antibiotics early during an ear infection contributes to recurrences, as well as bacterial resistance. Many of the doctors I have interviewed over the past decade have similar thoughts about antibiotic use.

"…I will prescribe an antibiotic when I feel it is called for, although I certainly try to avoid using them as much as possible," states Dr. Kenneth Bock. "Unlike most physicians, I will not prescribe an antibiotic without giving my patients probiotics…"

Prescriptions aren't our only source of antibiotics. The industrial usage of antibiotics in livestock feed is well-documented. This means that when we're ingesting animal products, we're also ingesting more antibiotics. Like their prescription counterparts, these secondary antibiotics contribute to antibiotic resistance and imbalanced intestinal flora.

Using probiotics with antibiotics

Lactic acid bacteria/probiotics help the body recover from overuse of antibiotics, whether they come from prescriptions and/or animal foods. Many healthcare professionals agree with Dr. Bock that probiotics must be used in conjunction with antibiotic treatment.

That's really the most important lesson we've learned about antibiotic use over the past decade. Never take an antibiotic without also taking a probiotic supplement. The antibiotic will still kill the bacteria and disrupt the balance for a time, but the probiotic will help replenish the good bacteria and promote proper bacterial balance.

Both clinical and controlled animal studies have shown that antibiotics reduce the very beneficial lactobacilli to low levels. However, within 24 hours of supplementation with probiotics, lactobacilli levels were restored.

In order to maximize the effectiveness of probiotic treatment, start taking the supplements as soon as possible. Continue for a minimum of seven to 14 days after antibiotic treatment has been completed. It is best to take the probiotics with meals, when antibiotics are not consumed.

Dr. Bock concludes, "Ideally, beneficial microorganisms like probiotics do no harm to the host, act against pathogens by means of several different mechanisms (thus minimizing the risk of the development of resistance), stimulate the host's defenses to destroy an invading pathogen, act promptly (unlike, for example, a vaccine), and aren't too expensive."

A 1996 article in the *Journal of the American Medical Association* (*JAMA*) sounded an alarm to healthcare professionals, asking them to consider new strategies for the treatment and prevention of infectious diseases. The use of probiotics is one of those strategies that deserves serious consideration among conventional healthcare professionals.

Common candidiasis

A negative, chronic by-product of antibiotic overuse is the overgrowth of *Candida albicans*, a fungi in the yeast family.

"Candida is one of the oldest surviving life forms, and it has had eons to perfect its adaptability," explains Dr. Bock.

When Candida overgrowth targets the vagina, it can cause vaginitis, or inflammation of the vagina. Vaginal candidiasis can become an acute, chronic problem for many women. It can even promote viral infections of the cervix. The female urogenital tract is sensitive to the good-versus-bad bacteria battle that similarly takes place in the intestines.

Fortunately, candidiasis, as well as other vaginal infections and associated problems, responds very favorably to probiotic treatment. One study involving 19 cases of non-specific infection of the vagina demonstrated a 95 percent cure rate using probiotics. The *American Journal of Obstetrics and Gynecology* reported the results of a much larger study of 444 patients with vaginitis. Ninety-two percent were cured and remained infection-free up to a year later.

"Several studies have correlated vaginal health (absence of infections) with the presence of lactobacilli…Some clinical substantiation of the ability of probiotics to decrease recurrence of urogenital infections in women exists," explains Dr. Mary Ellen Sanders in *Food Technology*. "Oral consumption of certain probiotic-containing products…was found to mediate decreased recurrence of Candida infections and bacterial vaginosis."

Women who experience chronic yeast infections can benefit greatly from probiotic supplements. Sometimes, yeast infections require an anti-fungal prescription. As in the case of antibiotics treatment, probiotics should also be used in conjunction with antifungal prescriptions to help preserve, enhance, and replenish good bacteria.

Dangerous diarrhea

One of the most common adverse effects of antibiotic therapy is known as antibiotic-associated diarrhea. It occurs in nearly 30 percent of all hospital patients and is associated with a three-fold risk of dying.

While we may think of diarrhea as merely an uncomfortable condition, it can become much more serious. In 1996, the World Health Organization reported that, of the most common infections worldwide, diarrheal diseases are the most prevalent with about 4 billion episodes in 1995. Of that number, more than 3 million deaths were attributed to various causes of diarrhea—most of them children.

As we learned earlier, water is removed from the food in the large intestine. By the time the substances we eat make their way through the colon to be removed, they should be solid. Diarrhea can result if the water is not removed while the material is in the large intestine, or if there is a bacterial infection or tumor in the colon, or if the lining of the colon becomes inflamed, causing blood, mucus, and other fluids to form in the stool.

In addition to producing watery stools, diarrhea may be accompanied by fever, thirst, nausea, pain, and cramping. Excessive diarrhea often results in dehydration. Children are especially vulnerable to diarrhea, since they cannot withstand dehydration as long as adults can. Among the numerous infections that cause infantile diarrhea, the most common throughout the world is due to rotavirus. Rotavirus accounts for about 20 to 40 percent of deaths in children less than five years old.

Diarrhea is the body's effort to eliminate unnecessary and harmful materials. Therefore, antidiarrheal drugs should be used with caution. Dr. Tomotari Mitsuoka points out that by using these medications, we keep those harmful materials inside the body. This worsens the root problem, and can actually delay recovery from the diarrhea.

Studies involving patients with diarrhea have demonstrated that probiotic supplementation significantly:

1. Changed the composition of the stool, making it more firm;
2. Reduced related symptoms associated with the condition;
3. Enhanced the immune system's response to the rotavirus.

Researchers have also confirmed that patients with non-bloody diarrhea usually have a deficiency of *Lactobacillus acidophilus*. It makes sense to supplement the diet with probiotics to help alleviate diarrhea and stimulate a positive immune response against the rotavirus.

NOTE: Diarrhea can be a very dangerous condition, especially in children. If there is blood in the stool, or the diarrhea has persisted for several days, see a qualified healthcare professional right away before complete dehydration occurs. Dehydration can be life-threatening.

Dangers in our food and water

How many times have you gone on vacation and heard: "Don't drink the water"? If you ignore this advice, you could end up with what has been called traveller's diarrhea. It's not a fun way to spend a hard-earned vacation.

How many times have you flipped through the newspaper, only to find another report of a *Salmonella* or *E. coli* outbreak? These reports have become almost commonplace. There was a time when such reports would send fear throughout the community. Today, we read the reports with a simple sigh of relief if the outbreak didn't affect us.

A pathogen is a microorganism capable of producing a disease. As previously mentioned, the existence of food- and water-borne pathogens has increased dramatically. Many epidemiologists say the problem is even more serious than most people realize.

Four of the most common causes of food-borne infections are:

1. *Salmonella*
2. *E. coli*
3. Staphylococcus
4. Listeria

These and other pathogens enter the body through our food and water, swinging their elbows and throwing around their weight. Their goal is to take over the "living space."

One of the first lines of defense against these pathogens is your internal microflora. The job of our resident friendly bacteria is to show these pathogens the door! If the good bacteria are compromised, of course the pathogens will have their way with us. Not only will the pathogens take up residence, they can also multiply. That makes it even more difficult for the good bacteria to keep them at bay. That's the bad news. The good news is that you can restore balance and order to your digestive system by taking probiotic supplements.

Pathogens can produce symptoms in as little as 15 minutes or as long as two weeks. Your system's response depends on which pathogen is at work and how healthy your internal ecosystem is. If your symptoms become severe or persist, you need to see a doctor.

Taking probiotics every day will help your GI tract defend against those sometimes not-so-subtle microbial attacks from whatever is consumed. At a bare minimum, it is always a good idea to take probiotics when travelling, or if you experience a bad reaction to something you ate or drank. For many of us, travelling includes a trip to the local health food store.

Relieving lactose intolerance

An important function of the small intestine is to metabolize lactose, a sugar substance found in milk and dairy products. With the help of the enzyme lactase, the small intestine is able to break down lactose into a usable form. Because of age or a genetic condition, many of us have a deficiency of the enzyme lactase. This condition is known as lactose intolerance. People who are lactose intolerant cannot break down lactose. Thus, lactose stays in the small intestine longer, causing fluid to build up. The unabsorbed particles then make their way to the large intestine, where they are joined with bacteria that cause gas, bloating, and discomfort.

Lactose intolerance is the most common genetic disorder in the world, afflicting half to two-thirds of the world's population. The first symptoms of lactose intolerance occur after a meal of lactose-containing foods, which are primarily dairy products. Within 20 to 30 minutes of consumption, a person with this condition can expect to experience abdominal discomfort, bloating, and maybe diarrhea. There may also be nausea, gas, audible bowel sounds, and cramping.

In severe cases of lactose intolerance, especially when it is undiagnosed in children, malabsorption of important nutrients can result from diarrhea. A child with lactose intolerance may also have difficulty gaining weight if dairy products are a part of the diet.

Avoidance of dairy products is the obvious treatment for individuals with this condition. Because yogurt is a fermented food, most of the milk lactose has been utilized by the bacteria used to make it. So, in many instances, it can be consumed on a lactose-intolerance diet. Some dairy products that contain the enzyme lactase are marketed specifically for people with lactose intolerance. If bone strength is an issue, lactose-intolerant individuals may want to take a comprehensive calcium/mineral supplement to offset the lack of calcium from dairy products. In addition, nutritional supplements containing the enzyme lactase can help individuals suffering from lactose intolerance.

Although I haven't heard much in the mass media, it is well documented that probiotics, specifically *Lactobacilli* and *Bifidobacteria*, can help ease the symptoms of lactose intolerance. These friendly bacteria help metabolize lactose in the small intestine, where it is supposed to be metabolized. This will reduce the amount of lactose moving into the large intestine, and help minimize the discomforts and dangers associated with lactose intolerance.

Cholesterol control
While you may have already heard about probiotic supplements for diarrhea or lactose intolerance, they are not often associated with cholesterol control. However, researchers have discovered that probiotics may play an important role in cholesterol metabolism and utilization. When you think about cholesterol, what pops into your head? While some people might picture their morning scrambled eggs, most people think of "danger." We've been trained to believe that cholesterol, in and of itself, is damaging. Yes, high cholesterol can contribute to heart disease. However, your body manufactures cholesterol for a reason—because you need it.

Cholesterol helps the body manufacture important adrenal and sex hormones. It is also required for proper nerve and brain function. Cholesterol even helps make vitamin D, an essential nutrient for strong bones.

As a nation, cholesterol levels are rising because of the consumption of too much fat and not enough fresh, unprocessed foods. Researchers have confirmed that high cholesterol levels can contribute to heart disease, the number-one killer disease in the United States, affecting more than 30 percent of the population.

According to the National Institutes of Health, about half a million people die each year from heart attacks. In the United States, 1.25 million heart attacks occur annually. Estimates show that a staggering one out of every two men aged 40 and younger, and one out of every three women, aged 40 and younger, will develop heart disease at some point in their lives. Obviously, heart disease is no longer a disease just affecting the elderly.

Clearly, controlling cholesterol levels is an important heart health goal. The famed Framingham Heart Study demonstrated that young adults with lower cholesterol levels have greater longevity and lower cardiovascular mortality. These results were confirmed recently in a report published in *JAMA.*

Estimates in 1994 by the National Institutes of Health (NIH) indicated that nearly 20 percent of the American population had high cholesterol. Recent estimates show that more than one-half of women over age 55 need to lower their cholesterol.

When considering your cholesterol levels, keep in mind that total cholesterol is not the main issue. We need to focus on the ratio of good to bad cholesterol. Low-density lipoprotein (LDL) is the bad cholesterol and high-density lipoprotein (HDL) is considered good. HDL transports fat in the blood to the liver, where it can be metabolized and then excreted. In contrast, LDL transports fat from the liver throughout the blood, where it can accumulate in the arteries, possibly leading to a heart attack.

Scientists have discovered that probiotics have a positive effect on cholesterol levels. While the exact mechanism of action is not known, 15 published studies since 1974, involving more than 500 people, have demonstrated that probiotics can significantly lower total cholesterol, as well as LDL (bad) cholesterol.

In addition, some preliminary studies involving high blood pressure have also been positive. Animal and some small human trials have produced a small, but statistically significant decrease in cases of mild hypertension.

NOTE: Do not stop taking a prescription medication without first consulting with your physician.

The cancer question

Cancer is one of the most feared diseases of our time. It remains one of the most expensive, deadly, and complex conditions known.

Almost any cell in our body can turn cancerous. There are hundreds of different types of cancers. Some are so virulent they can adapt to nearly every internal scenario and external assault.

Conventional medicine has tried to cut out these cancers with surgery, burn them out with radiation, and poison them with chemotherapy. The horrifying by-product of these options is that the radiation and chemotherapy can also kill the healthy cells—the ones that are trying to kill the cancer for us. Side effects of these treatments can be devastating. While the intention of this book is not to provide a complete description of cancer therapies, anyone with a cancer history or cancer diagnosis should be aware of the research on probiotics.

Growing evidence suggests a localized positive effect of probiotics for cancers of the digestive system. Both laboratory and human studies have shown that probiotics can counteract cancer growth in the colon and other sites within the digestive system.

Published results of a study in 1992, by researchers Aso and Akazan, demonstrated an increase in the recurrence-free period among patients with bladder cancer who took a probiotic supplement. In other research, stomach cancer patients who took probiotics remained cancer-free longer.

Recent studies have also involved a specific cancer-causing substance known as N-Nitrosodimethylamine (NDMA). It is thought that NDMA is formed in the GI tract and that bad bacteria may contribute to its formation. Because chronic renal failure patients cannot excrete metabolic waste such as this, they accumulate significant levels of NDMA in their blood. Consequently, they were used as a study group.

When the renal failure patients were taking lactobacilli supplements daily, their blood levels of NDMA were significantly reduced. More importantly, when the treatment stopped, the higher levels of NDMA rapidly returned. Certainly, lactobacilli supplementation contributed to the reduction in blood levels of this carcinogen.

It has been predicted that cancer will soon surpass heart disease as the number-one killer disease in the United States. There is no doubt that cancer has proven to be a tough opponent. Perhaps one day we will confirm that probiotics are an effective weapon we can use in our comprehensive attack against this devastating disease.

Chapter Four

Choosing and Using Probiotics

As we have learned, probiotics are powerful tools we can use to support good health. They can help prevent and treat a variety of illnesses. So, it may seem appropriate to run to the store and buy a probiotic supplement and begin taking it as soon as possible. Hold on—not so fast. I wish it were that easy. Unfortunately, choosing and using the proper probiotic supplement requires additional direction. Probiotic supplements are not equally effective.

This section will provide some general guidelines, as well as answers to commonly asked questions on this topic. I have relied on the expertise of healthcare experts, along with the information in the scientific literature, to help answer any remaining questions you may have, and to help clarify some points that may still be confusing.

Begin at the beginning

It has been said that the end product is only as good as the beginning material. This is definitely the case with probiotics. To get the best, most effective probiotics supplement, you need to find out where the friendly bacteria actually came from.

One of the most important aspects of probiotics is that these friendly bacteria need to attach to the intestinal wall. This is known as implantation. Once they find their "niche," they can easily grow, multiply, and achieve much greater numbers than those "passing through," or not attached. A number of lab studies have shown that bacteria from human sources attach to cells up to 10 times greater than dairy bacteria.

While many studies demonstrate the benefits of dairy-based bacteria, these effects don't appear to last as long as human-based bacteria. Innovative research using human strains has uncovered more effective ways to achieve optimum implantation.

Utilizing human strain bacteria from healthy human volunteers, scientists were and are able to isolate and replicate the good bacteria in your GI tract. This is a critical point to remember. Research has confirmed that human strain bacteria that have been colonized and purified using state-of-the-art technology are more likely to thrive in the human intestinal tract than non-human strains. It makes sense, doesn't it?

Most probiotic supplements on the market today come from dairy products, which originated as fortuitous contaminants in fresh milk. As I mentioned before, many researchers contend that these milk-based bacteria are less likely to "stick" and grow than human strain bacteria.

As you know, acidophilus and bifidobacteria are normal residents of the GI tract in humans. Some of the strains used to culture yogurt, however, are not present in human microflora and do not implant and colonize. If there is no colonization, there are not enough friendly bacteria to do the job.

In addition, researchers have found that certain yogurt strains may not resist stomach acid, and never make the trip to the lower intestines. This too is extremely critical. In order for the bacteria to stick, they must first bypass the stomach. From there, we want them to move into the colon and stay for awhile so they can fortify the good bacteria already there.

Human strains have been shown to resist stomach acid when consumed with food. These bacteria are already used to the environment of the human intestinal tract and are more likely to survive and colonize. Remember, there is power in numbers.

One human strain of bacteria has been used for more than 30 years by more than 30,000 hospitals and clinics throughout the world. Countless individuals have benefitted from these potent probiotics.

While the source of the bacteria is a big issue, it is not the only confusing aspect of probiotics. The most important factor in a probiotics supplement is the stability of the bacterial strains. Probiotics are live cells. Therefore, if the manufacturing process is inadequate, the bacteria may already be activated in the product. If they are already activated, they are useless to the consumer. In contrast, a high-quality, human strain probiotics supplement can remain stable, at room temperature, until the time of expiration. It is not activated until you take it, so you get the benefit of live cells.

Let's take a closer look at the different questions I have received over the years. You just may see yourself in some of these questions and benefit from the answers.

Q. I find the dosage amounts confusing. Please explain what these numbers mean, and what potency I should look for in a probiotic supplement.

It's not surprising that this area is confusing to most people. Bacteria are numbered in millions, billions, and trillions. Those numbers are difficult to fathom.

"Billion" is the word to remember. That's 1,000,000,000 (10^9). According to specialists in the field, the minimum number of viable bacteria needed is at least 10^8 or 10^9, or one-half to one billion per serving. This is the suggested minimum. More can be taken. In some clinical studies involving infants, for example, as many as 10^{12} have been taken without side effects.

supplementwatch.com has reported its test results on the probiotics products on the market. According to the report, only one product has the live cells claimed on the product label. All the other products fall short.

Remember, just because the label says there are a billion bacteria at packaging doesn't necessarily mean that there are a billion when you buy them or after a month on the shelf. The key is to become familiar with the probiotic manufacturer. Choose a product from a manufacturer with a history of producing probiotic supplements and a strong reputation in the natural health industry.

Check the probiotic label for the statement, "One billion live cells *prior to expiration date*." Many probiotic labels feature the meaningless statement, "One billion live cells *at the time of manufacture.*" After these probiotic supplements are manufactured, live cells may die quickly due to the instability of their bacteria, even in the refrigerator.

Q. I was told that I should take an acidophilus supplement early in the morning on an empty stomach, when stomach acid is low. What is your view on this?

The issue of stomach acid is an important one. We agree that stomach acid can destroy the probiotics and cause you to waste your time and hard-earned money. There are few strains of bacteria that can withstand the strong acids that are produced on an empty stomach for extended periods of time.

After a meal, the stomach becomes less acidic. This allows bacteria a better chance of surviving. In several studies, survival of *Lactobacillus acidophilus* was found to be much lower in participants who were fasting versus participants who were fed. In addition, the decreased acidity following the consumption of food enabled the population of *Bifidobacterium* to double in size.

Therefore, I recommend that you take your probiotic supplement with food or shortly after eating.

Q. With all the different strains and confusing names, what types of bacteria should I look for in a product?

I believe the two most important strains of friendly bacteria are *Lactobacillus acidophilus* and *Bifidobacterium*. These bacteria will provide benefit throughout the intestinal tract. In the healthy human, *Lactobacillus acidophilus* bacteria exist from the upper part of the small intestine to the lower part of the small intestine. *Bifidobacterium* exist from the lower part of the small intestine to the large intestine. By combining these strains, you should be able to suppress harmful bacteria and toxic substances along the entire intestinal tract.

Also, I recommend human strain probiotics that are stable at room temperature for their full shelf live.

Q. I eat a very healthful diet. Do I really need to take probiotic supplements?

Congratulations for paying close attention to diet. That's really the foundation of overall optimum health and vitality. We must always first try to get all we need from diet, and then supplement from there. After all, that's why they are called "dietary supplements" in the first place.

Unfortunately, even someone meticulous about diet cannot overcome these common barriers to good health:

• Toxins and chemicals in our air, water, and food.
• Food processing, preservatives, colorings, and hidden antibiotics.
• Second-hand tobacco smoke.
• Recycled air on an airplane.
• Interaction with people who may be carriers of viruses and bacteria.

However, let's not get paranoid. Healthy immune and digestive systems can help us battle just about anything. The key is to give those systems as much power as possible.

You may not feel you need to take probiotics all the time. However, I do suggest frequent courses of probiotic supplements to ensure a balanced internal ecosystem. It is impossible to determine exactly when you will need them. That's why I take them on a daily basis.

Here is what I recommend. You should supplement with probiotics every day if:

1. You have a family history of cancer, heart disease, or digestive problems (including lactose intolerance).
2. You are over the age of 55 or you experience significant stress.
3. You are a frequent traveller—even domestically.

Whether you travel for business or pleasure, you should supplement prior, during, and after your trip(s). Finally, and very important, **when you take antibiotics, you should take probiotics**.

Q. I was always under the impression that acidophilus supplements need to be refrigerated once they are open. What is your view on this?

The vast majority of probiotics need to be refrigerated, which is why you usually find them in the refrigerated section of the store. However, some manufacturers have perfected their processing so the bacteria are stable, some even for years, at room temperature. I prefer these because they are convenient to take along when travelling. Also, because they need no refrigeration, the actual number of viable bacteria have been shown to be exceptionally stable over time. That ensures that we are getting what the label says is there.

The key to friendly bacteria's effectiveness is their ability to revive once they enter a liquid environment. This ability to survive and thrive largely depends on how healthy they were before they were dried and how they were dried. Human strain cultures from Japan are cultured and then dried using a unique method that allows them to stay dormant for more than three years, even when kept at room temperature. In contrast, most products on the shelf are viable for less than a few months at the most.

Moisture is the main threat to acidophilus viability. Refrigerating an acidophilus bottle can result in condensation, which results in a lack of viability. For this reason, probiotics should not be refrigerated.

Q. Can I build up a resistance to probiotics, making them ineffective if I take them every day?

No, you cannot build up a resistance to probiotic supplements. In fact, because your body is constantly eliminating bacteria, it is important to replenish the good bacteria on a daily basis.

Q. Should I worry about taking probiotics with other medications? If I am taking antibiotics, for example, should I wait to start taking probiotics after the antibiotics are done?

If you are taking antibiotics, you should also take probiotics, but at different times of the day. Take your probiotic supplement during or right after a meal, and that you take your antibiotic at a different time during the day. Taking the probiotic with the evening meal may be best so that the good bacteria have at least eight hours to colonize before you take your antibiotic again. It is always best to take the probiotic supplement for at least two weeks, even after you are done with your antibiotic prescription. Some strains of friendly bacteria are resistant to various antibiotics, so they may colonize and provide benefit even while you are taking the antibiotic.

I am not aware of any medications that should not be taken with probiotics. However, if you have a weakened immune system, it is always best to discuss your supplement program with your medical doctor.

Q. Do the dead bacteria in our systems pose any risk? Are probiotic supplements safe?

Based on the information that is presently available, there is no reason to believe dead bacteria will do us any harm. That makes sense. After all, we have been ingesting milk-based bacteria and bacteria from other fermented products for generations. In fact, some studies have demonstrated that dead, friendly bacteria are still somewhat capable of supporting the immune system and enhancing resistance to pathogens like *E. coli*. However, the dead friendly bacteria are not capable of competing with or killing bad bacteria. Therefore, live friendly bacteria are the best choice.

Probiotic supplements are very safe, even for women who are pregnant or lactating. However, if you are pregnant, check with your doctor before taking probiotics or any other supplement.

Consider the following study that confirms the safety of probiotics: A multi-strain probiotic, containing *Lactobacillus acidophilus* and *Bifidobacterium bifidum,* was administered to 180 individuals from eight different medical facilities. The period of administration ranged from two days to several weeks. At the conclusion of the trial, none of the participants reported any problems associated with probiotic use. Additional safety data have also indicated an absence of side effects from lactic acid bacteria products.

Q. When can I expect to notice a difference in my health after I start using probiotics?

That depends. If you are fairly healthy and are using probiotics to prevent disease, you will notice a difference in the absence of illness and an enhanced vitality. The effect will be subtle. It's not like taking an aspirin and getting relief from your headache in 20 minutes, or taking a sleeping pill and becoming drowsy shortly thereafter. While the effect may not be as dramatic, probiotics work in an important, long-lasting way.

It is important to depend on the scientific data that clearly establish the benefits of probiotics. However, the results that everyday people experience are also important. Over the years, I have heard many stories from people who have had remarkable results with probiotics. Here are just a few things I have heard:

- "I normally get bloated after I eat but then I take these [human strain probiotics] and I don't get bloated. I was amazed."
  —A.W., Dunedin, FL

- "I had an infection with *C. difficile* and was placed on an antibiotic. I got so sick from the medication that I stopped taking it when a friend recommended probiotics. The probiotic supplement kicked the *C. difficile* within two weeks with no side effects. It was a life saver to me."
  —Mrs. J., Jacksonville, FL

• "My wife suffered from quite a bit of digestive discomfort. Everything had failed, including frequent attempts with over-the-counter and prescription medications. Within a few days of taking [human strain probiotics], her problems subsided. Until you've been through the pain, it is difficult to appreciate a product that brings such immediate and consistent relief."

—M.S., Austin, TX

• "I have had ulcerative colitis my whole life...acidophilus has helped keep it under control."

—W.S., Detroit, MI

• "It [human strain probiotic product] helps control my stomach bloating and elimination."

—J.S., LA

• "[The human strain probiotic supplement] seems to be helping with my irritable bowel syndrome. It helps to harden the stools. I had diarrhea and it helped."

—E.W.G., Tallahasse, FL

• "Since 1994 I have had problems of bloating and gas. I was diagnosed first with irritable bowel syndrome and now they have discovered that it is really Crohn's disease. After taking [human strain probiotic], 90 percent of my symptoms have been relieved."

—T.B., Concord, CA

• "I normally get thrush and yeast infections when on antibiotics. I have had a real problem with bronchitis. After I started taking the antibiotic this time I took [human strain probiotics]. I didn't get a yeast infection or have a problem with thrush."

—C.H., Leavenworth, KS

- "…I was telling my friend who is a pharmacist about my stomach problems. He is the person that told me to stop taking antacids and try [human strain probiotics]. I've been taking [human strain probiotics] for about a month and all of my stomach problems seemed to have disappeared. My stomach has calmed down and my infrequent bouts of nausea have gone away."

—S.R.S., NY

- "While working with my naturopathic physician to determine if candida was the cause of my food allergies, a stool sample revealed that I had large amounts of yeast and no *Lactobacillus* in spite of the fact that I had been consistently taking an acidophilus supplement. I switched to a human strain probiotic supplement. Six weeks later, the stool sample showed no yeast and a maximum *Lactobacillus* count. This result convinced me to recommend the new product to my customers who are looking for a probiotic supplement."

—V.W.
Vivianne's Health Foods, BC, Canada

- "Eight years ago I was overdosed with antibiotics in treatment for a ganglious condition. Acquired *Lichen planus* as a result, a disease caused by antibiotic overdose. Been to many doctors. Affected all mucous membranes, ears (had to wear two hearing aids), vaginal area, and mouth. Lost my hair and some of my fingernails. Had a sore on right cheek for probably 18 years and could not heal it. Was taking steroids to deal with sores in mouth. Within one week of taking [human strain probiotics], mouth was noticeably better, and within 2 weeks even the redness in the sore spot was disappearing…Tried acidophilus before but got no effect at all even taking for 30 days."

—E.G., MO

• "After a trip to Mexico, I was diagnosed with amobic dysentery. Since then, I have had constant problems with diarrhea and irritable bowel syndrome (IBS). For the past 14 months, I have been on and off antibiotics. I have had constant infections and intestinal and urinary problems. After I started taking [human strain probiotics], within three days, all of my IBS symptoms disappeared. I consider this a miracle product. It has literally saved my life."

—C.C., Valpraiso, IN

Q. Are human strain probiotics safe for animals?

Definitely. In fact, some of our most successful testimonials are from people giving probiotics to their pets. Listen to this story:

"I recently had a three-pound Pomeranian pick up a virus and couldn't control the diarrhea. I opened two capsules of the probiotic supplement on a bit of baby food. She didn't seem to mind the taste. She is now fat and happy again and trying to rule the roost (all three pounds of her!). Before giving her the probiotics, I was unsuccessful at stabilizing the bowel and stomach. After I got the probiotics in her, she settled down."

—T.D., Westminster, MD
Pomeranian Club of Greater Baltimore

As a general rule, probiotics will benefit animals the same way they benefit humans. They will also help alleviate the same illnesses in animals as they do in humans. Probiotics are very safe and effective for our four-legged friends.

Chapter Five

The Probiotics Plan

The topic of probiotics can be complex and confusing. This is not surprising considering that the digestive system is one of the most complicated systems of the human body. In addition, the bacteria that inhabit this system can be difficult to understand due to their intricate make-up and large numbers.

The flurry of activity that takes place in our internal bacterial world can be difficult to describe and even more challenging to understand. However, beneath all of this complexity lie some basic facts.

Scientific research has indicated that these vast numbers of bacteria help us stay alive. Ideally, we can live in harmony with both the good and bad bacteria. Probiotics provide us with both a protective and therapeutic tool we can use to gain vital health and prevent illness. As we have learned, most of us are well served by adding human strain probiotics to our supplement regimen. Probiotics are ideal for individuals who:

- are taking antibiotics;
- travel frequently;
- have a history of cancer, high cholesterol, or heart disease;
- are under emotional and/or physical stress;
- frequently experience constipation or diarrhea;
- are lactose intolerant; and
- are inactive and have an unhealthy diet.

Because friendly bacteria continually die off, they need to be replenished. For this reason, I believe a probiotic should be taken like you would a multivitamin/mineral supplement—on a daily basis. Let's review the other important issues described in this book.

Seven most commonly asked questions and answers

1. What are probiotics? Probiotics are organisms that help improve the environment of the intestinal tract. They help restore balanced numbers of known beneficial bacteria to create a healthier internal environment.

2. Why should you take probiotics? When we don't have enough friendly bacteria, we can get sick. We know that various factors can disrupt our intestinal bacterial balance. These factors include:

- Antibiotic use
- Travelling (domestic and international)
- Physical and psychological stress
- Pathogens (i.e., microorganisms such as bacteria and fungus that cause disease) in the food, water, or air
- Change in diet
- Aging

Probiotics can help restore balanced numbers of friendly bacteria, creating a healthier environment in the intestinal tract. In this way, they protect against diarrhea, constipation, and other uncomfortable intestinal symptoms.

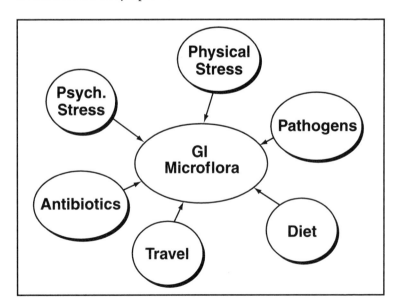

3. What are the two most common strains of probiotics and where are they distributed? *Lactobacillus acidophilus* is distributed in the upper and lower small intestine; *Bifidobacterium* is distributed in the lower small intestine and the large intestine. Combining these two strains can protect the complete intestinal tract.

4. What is the overall effect of probiotics? Probiotic supplements help stimulate a variety of important, health-improving activities, including:

• Production of substances, such as natural acids (e.g., lactic acid, acetic acid) and antimicrobial factors, that suppress the growth of harmful bacteria.

• Activation of immune cells, such as macrophages.

• Production of B vitamins and enzymes (e.g., lactase for lactose digestion).

• Recycling of toxins and decrease in their absorption (e.g., nitrosamines and other cancer-causing substances).

• Possible reduction of cholesterol absorption.

Toxins can damage the liver. Furthermore, once they bypass the liver's filter function, they cause problems throughout the body.

5. What strain of probiotic supplement is best and why? We recommend room-temperature, stable human strain bacteria for the following reasons:

• They are pre-adapted for growth in the human intestinal tract.

• They are able to withstand the acidity of the stomach when food is present.

• They are able to withstand bile and other compounds in the intestinal tract.

• They are able to adhere ("stick") to the cells lining the intestinal tract, and can work there.

• They stay alive at room temperature and do not require refrigeration.

6. What is the proper amount of bacteria necessary for effectiveness? Experts agree that the minimum daily requirement is between one-half to one billion *live* cells per day. Exact dosage, however, has not been established. There is presently no government recommended dietary allowance (RDA) for probiotics. Several clinical studies have demonstrated good results from the use of 1 billion live cells.

7. Should you take probiotics on an empty stomach or with food? Probiotics should be taken with food for the following reasons:
- Few strains of bacteria can withstand the harsh acidity of an empty stomach.
- Food dilutes stomach acid to levels bacteria can withstand.
- Fewer bacteria have been shown to survive in fasted than in fed subjects.
- Food enhances survival and growth of bacteria.

Final thoughts

With the countless brands and types of probiotics on the market, it can be difficult to choose the best supplement. Follow these strict guidelines when choosing a probiotic supplement:
- Buy a brand from a manufacturer with a solid reputation and a history of producing quality probiotics. These products should be backed by solid stability study results during their entire shelf life. Ask the manufacturer whether these studies support the particular product.
- Choose a brand that contains cultured human strain bacteria and that does not need to be refrigerated. Remember, refrigeration can cause condensation and the resulting moisture can destroy the bacteria.
- Don't purchase based on price. You could be wasting your money, and even more importantly, valuable time.
- Ask about the science. The human strain, room-temperature, stable bacteria that I mention in this book are supported by many clinical and laboratory scientific studies.

It is important to choose a quality probiotic supplement in order to gain the health benefits. I use probiotic supplements every day to consistently replenish the supply of good bacteria. As a preventive, probiotic supplements can be an important addition to your supplement regimen.

If you do not use probiotics daily, you may want to consider them specifically for the following conditions/situations:

- **A weakened immune system.** More evidence is needed to confirm the broad range of benefits of probiotics for the immune system. However, scientific studies show that probiotics can activate immune cells, increase natural killer cell activity, and stimulate a greater immune response.
- **Antibiotic use.** Probiotics help alleviate the symptoms associated with antibiotic use by replenishing the friendly bacteria that many antibiotics kill.
- **Vaginal candidiasis.** This is a key side effect of chronic antibiotic use. When taken with antimycotics (i.e., antifungal medications), probiotics can help alleviate this problem.
- **Diarrhea and constipation.** Probiotics are good for intestinal symptoms, such as diarrhea and constipation, that are caused by a deficiency of good bacteria. They are especially effective against rotavirus, which causes diarrhea and accounts for 20 to 40 percent of deaths in children younger than five years old.
- **Food and water pathogens.** Probiotics help prevent symptoms associated with food and/or water contaminants. This is why probiotics are so important for travellers.
- **Lactose intolerance.** Probiotics can help the digestive system produce the enzyme lactase. Lactase is deficient in individuals with lactose intolerance, one of the most common genetic disorders in the world.
- **High cholesterol.** Preliminary studies indicate that probiotics can possibly reduce cholesterol absorption, thereby helping to control high cholesterol.
- **Cancer.** Probiotics have been shown to reduce the absorption of cancer-causing substances such as nitrosamines.

Probiotics are an exciting area of study. Sophisticated scientific techniques, combined with an elevated level of interest from the medical community, will make this an interesting topic to follow. Based on my experience with probiotics, it is rewarding to see the countless people who have benefited from utilizing probiotic supplements. I am confident that number will continue to swell as more uses for these friendly bacteria are uncovered.

Resources/Recommended Reading

INTERNET:

www.impakt.com = information about IMPAKT Communications and
    the information and books published by IMPAKT

www.probiotics.com = information about human strain probiotics

www.questvitamins.com = information about the quality products manufactured
    and distributed by Quest Vitamins of Canada

www.wakunaga.com = information about the quality products manufactured
    and distributed by Wakunaga of America

www.supplementwatch.com = ratings and warnings about nutritional
    supplements

www.kyolic.com

BOOKS AND PUBLICATIONS:

The Road to Immunity by Kenneth Bock, M.D., and Nellie Sabin,
    Pocket Books, New York, NY, 1997

Activate Your Immune System by Leonid Ber, M.D., and Karolyn A. Gazella,
    IMPAKT, Green Bay, WI, 1998

Bergey's Manual of Determinative Bacteriology, Ninth Edition by
    William Hensyl, Williams & Wilkins, 1994

Bergey's Manual of Systemic Bacteriology, Volume 2 by Peter Sneath,
    Nicholas Mair, Elizabeth Sharpe, and John Holt, Williams & Wilkins, 1986

Complete Candida Yeast Guidebook by Jeanne Marie Martin with
    Zoltan Rona, M.D., Prima, Rocklin, CA, 1996

Lactic Acid Bacteria by Seppo Salminen and Atte vonWright,
    Marcell Dekker, Inc., 1993

Probiotics: The Scientific Basis by Roy Fuller, Chapman & Hall, London, 1992

References

1. Anonymous: The influence of feeding cultured products on the microbial ecology of the gut. *International Dairy Federation Bulletin* 159: 5. In: Human Colonic Bacteria. (Gibson G.R. and Macfarlane G.T. eds.) pp. 261. CRC Press, 1995.

2. Arita M., Honda T and Miwatani T: Bacteriological study of lactic acid bacteria with multiple resistance. *Journal of Infectious Diseases* 60(3): 239, 1986.

3. Ballongue J: Bifidobacteria and probiotic action. In: *Lactic Acid Bacteria*. (Salminen, S. and Wright, A.V. ed.) Ch. 13. pp. 365, 409. Marcel Dekker Inc., New York, 1993.

4. Berrada N, Larochye G, Lemeland JF, and Tonetti H: Survie de bifidobactéries dans L'estomac de l'homme, in Les laits Fermentés. Actualité de la Recherche. John Libbey Eurotext, pp. 259-260. From: *Lactic Acid Bacteria* (Salminen, S. and Wright, A. V. ed.) p. 408. Marcel Dekker Inc., New York, 1993.

5. Calicchia ML, Wang CIE, Nomura T, Yotsuzuka F, and Osato DW: Selective enumeration of Bifidobacterium bifidum, Enterococcus faecium, and Streptomycin-Resistant Lactobacillus acidophilus from a Mixed Probiotic Product. *Journal of Food Protection* 56(11): 954-957, 1993.

6. Conway PL, Gorbach SL, and Golden BR: Survival of lactic acid bacteria in the human stomach and adhesion to intestinal cells. *Journal of Dairy Science* 70:1-12, 1987.

7. Deguchi Y, Morishita T, and Mutai M: Comparative studies on synthesis of water-soluble vitamins among human species of bifidobacteria. *Agric Biol Chem* 49(1): 13-19, 1985.

8. *Food Chemicals Codex., Third Edition.* Food and Nutrition Board. Nutrition Research Council. National Academy Press, Washington D.C. pp.108-109, 1981.

9. Goldin BR and Gorbach SL: Alterations of the intestinal microflora by diet, oral antibiotics, and lactobacillus: Decreased production of free amines from aromatic nitro compounds, azo dyes, and glucoronides. *JNCL* 73(3): 689-695, 1984.

10. Goldin BR and Gorbach SL: Probiotics for humans. In: *Probiotics. The Scientific Basis* (Fuller, R., ed.), Ch. 13, pp. 367-368. Chapman & Hall, London, 1992.

11. Goldin BR and Gorbach SL: Probiotics for humans. In: *Probiotics. The Scientific Basis* (Fuller, R., ed.), Ch. 13, p. 366. Chapman & Hall, London, 1992.

12. Goldin BR and Gorbach SL: Probiotics for humans. In: *Probiotics. The Scientific Basis* (Fuller, R., ed.), Ch. 13, pp. 361-362, 369. Chapman & Hall, London, 1992.

13. Hammer HF: Colonic hydrogen absorption: quantification of its effect on hydrogen accumulation caused by bacterial fermentation of carbohydrates. *Gut* 34: 818-822, 1992.

14. Hatcher GE and Lambrecht RS: Augmentation of macrophage phagocytic activity by cell-free extracts of selected lactic acid-producing bacteria. *J Dairy Sci* 76(9): 2485-2492, 1993.

15. Havenaar R, Ten Brink B and In'T Veld JHJ: Probiotics for humans. In: *Probiotics. The Scientific Basis* (Fuller, R., ed.), Ch. 9, p. 215. Chapman & Hall, London, 1992.

16. Honma N: Intestinal bacteria flora of infants and infection protection. *Pediatric Clinics* 27(11): 20, 1974.

17. Honma N: On effects of lactic acid bacteria. Part I Biological significance. *New Medicines and Clinics* 35(12): 2687-2695, 1986.

18. Honma N, Ohtani K, and Kikuchi H: On effects of lactic acid bacteria. Part II. Clinical effects. *New Medicines and Clinics* 36(1): 75, 1987.

19. Iwama T: Resistance of lactic acid bacteria products (Streptococcus Faecalis) against artificial gastric acid and a number of anti-bacteria. *Pharmacy* 21(5): 69, 1970.

20. Katagiri S: Study on anti-diarrhea effects. *Basics and Clinics* 20(17): 651-653, 1986.

21. Kawai K, Ida K, Seo T, Wakabayashi T, Kakutanik H, Matsuda I, Uematsu H, Taniguchi M, and Takato, H: Basic research study and treatment of peptic ulcer (Stomach pH after meals). *Clinics and Research* 44(4): 104, 1967.
22. Kochar N, Mehta A, Abraham P, and Bhatt R: In vitro effect of lactobacilli on intestinal anaerobic flora and intestinal gas. *Microecol Ther* 19: 119-120. In: *Lactic Acid Bacteria* (Salminen, S. and Wright, A. V. ed.) p. 207. Marcel Dekker Inc., New York, 1993.
23. Lichtenstein AH and Golden BR: Lactic acid bacteria and intestinal drug and cholesterol metabolism. In: *Lactic Acid Bacteria* (Salminen, S. and Wright, A.V. ed.) Ch. 8, pp. 232-233. Marcel Dekker Inc., New York, 1993.
24. Mccann T, Egan T, and Weber GH: Assay procedures for commercial probiotic cultures. *Journal of Food Protection* 59(1): 41-45, 1996.
25. Mitsuoka T: Important discovery: aging was stopped by intestine. *Seishun Shuppan-Sha*, Tokoyo, Japan, 1991.
26. Mitsuoka T: *Intestinal Bacteria and Health: An Introductory Narrative*. Harcourt Brace, Jovanovich Japan, Inc., Tokyo, 1978.
27. Mitsuoka T: Intestinal bacteria flora and its significance. *Clinics and Bacteria* 2(3): 55-97, 1975.
28. Mitsuoka T: Bacteria in the Intestines. *Medicina* 21(8): 1374., 1984
29. Mitsuoka T: Effect of lactic acid bacteria and new application areas. *Journal of Japan Food Industry* 31(4): 285, 1984.
30. Murphy EL and Colloway DH: The effect of antibiotic drugs on the volume and composition of the intestinal gas from beans. *American Journal of Digestive Disorders* 17: 639-642, 1972.
31. Nakamura H, Murakami R, Hayano M, and Matsuo T: Change of faeces bacteria flora during administration of aminobenzyl penicillin and effect of use of Biofermin R. *Pediatric Clinics* 35(10): 128, 1982.
32. On intestinal bacteria flora. Interview with Prof. Emeritus N. Honma of Dokkyo Medical College. *Pharmacology News* (8): 21, 1987.
33. Parker RB: Probiotics: Production, efficiency, and animal health. *Microbiologie Aliments Nutrition* 2:371-377, 1984.
34. Parker RB: Probiotics, the other half of the antibiotics story. *Animal Nutrition & Health*, 1974.
35. Perman JA, Modler S, and Olson AC: Role of pH in production of hydrogen from carbohydrates by colonic bacterial flora. *Journal of Clinical Investigation* 67: 643-650, 1981.
36. Prochaska LJ and Piekutowski WV *Med. Hypothesis* 42: 355-362, 1994.
37. Robins-Brown RM and Levine M: The fate of ingested lactobacilli in the proximal small intestine. *American Journal of Clinical Nutrition* 34:514-519, 1981.
38. Salminen S, Deighton M and Gorbach S: Lactic acid bacteria in health and disease. In: *Lactic Acid Bacteria*. (Salminen, S. and Wright, A.V. ed.) Ch. 7, pp. 200-201. Marcel Dekker Inc., New York, 1993.
39. Sanders ME: Probiotics. *Food Technology* 53:11, November 1999.
40. Weber G, Parker RB: Lactobacilli and human health. *Pharm Alert* 4:1, April 1997.
41. Whitney CG, et. al: Increasing prevalence of multidrug-resistant streptococcus pneumoniae in the United States. *The New England Journal of Medicine* 343:26, December 28, 2000.
42. Yamamoto T, Kishida Y, Ishida T and Hanedano M: Effect of lactic acid bacteria on intestinally decomposed substance producing bacteria of human source. *Basics and Clinics* 20(14): 123, 1986.
43. Yamashita M, Fujisaki M, Ohkushi E, Kaihatsu K and Uchida S: Ecological study of effects of administration of three kinds of lactic acid bacteria on suppression of intestinal decomposed substance. *Clinics and Microorganisms* 13(b): 87, 1987.
44. Yoneda K: Biological study on live bacteria products in the market. *Medicine and Pharmacology* 17(6): 1529-1534, 1987.

Other booklets/books published by IMPAKT Communications, Inc.:

Booklets

• *Dealing with Diabetes: Effective Herbal Solution* by Leonid Ber, M.D., and Frances E. FitzGerald
• *Digestion and Detox: Traditional Herbal Remedies Provide Ultimate Protection* by Leonid Ber, M.D., and Frances E. FitzGerald
• *Discover the Power of Aged Garlic Extract* by Rowan Hamilton, M.N.I.M.H, and Arnold Fox, M.D.
• *Protecting the Prostate* by Jean-Yves Dionne, B.Sc., Phm., and Karolyn A. Gazella
• *The Secret of St. John's Wort Revealed: Hyperforin for Depression* by Jean-Yves Dionne, B.Sc., Phm., and Sherry Torkos, B.Sc., Phm.
• *Superior Healing Power of SAMe* by Sherry Torkos, B.Sc., Phm., and Karolyn A. Gazella
• *Vanish Varicose Veins with Horse Chestnut Seed Extract* by Sherry Torkos, B.Sc., Phm.
• *Winning at Weight Loss: Achieve Healthy, Permanent Results* by Sherry Torkos, B.Sc., Phm., and Frances E. FitzGerald
• *Your Child's Health: Natural Solutions to Common Ailments* by Angela Stengler, N.D., and Mark Stengler, N.D.

Books

• *Activate Your Immune System* by Leonid Ber, M.D., and Karolyn A. Gazella
• *Build Bone Health: Prevent and Treat Osteoporosis* by Freedolf Anderson, M.D.
• *Buyer Be Wise! The Consumer's Guide to Buying Quality Nutritional Supplements* by Karolyn A. Gazella
• *Devour Disease with Shark Liver Oil* by Peter T. Pugliese, M.D., with John Heinerman, Ph.D.
• *Menopause Naturally* by Kathleen Frye, M.D., and Claudia Wingo, R.N.

These booklets and books are available at your local health food store or by calling (800) 477-2995 (credit card orders only). www.impakt.com

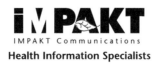

iMPAKT
IMPAKT Communications
Health Information Specialists

www.impakt.com